IMPROVE YOUR CHART READING SKILLS

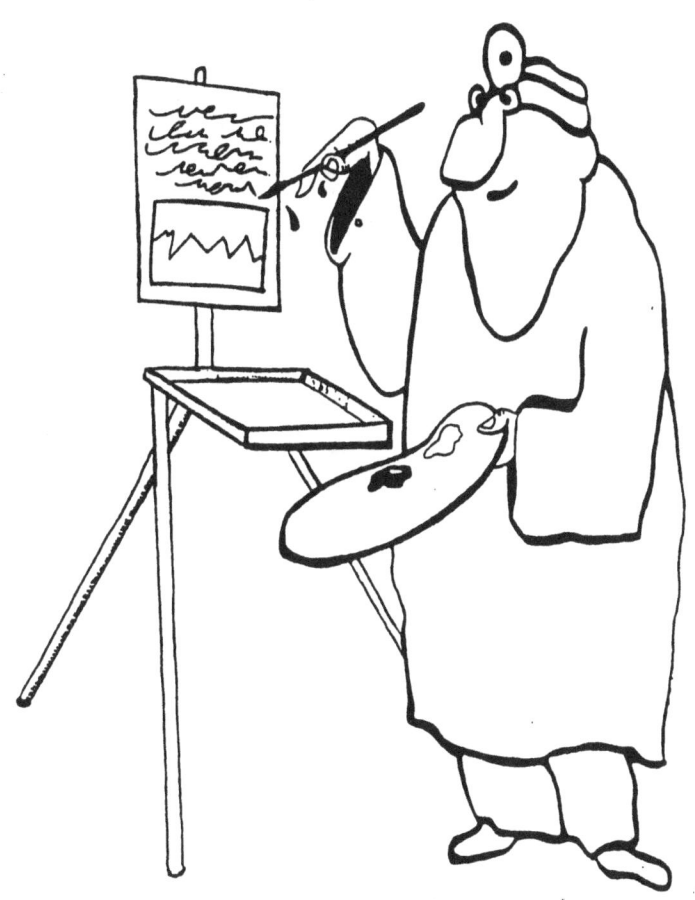

I. Wright Badlee, M.D.
Hugh Kant Reed, M.D.
Ida Cyper Scribbles, RN

IMPROVE YOUR CHART READING SKILLS

FIRST EDITION
Copyright ©2001 by Malcom S. Rosenberg

All rights reserved. No part of this publication may be reproduced, stored in a retrieval system or transmitted, in any form or by any means, electronic, mechanical, photocopying, recording, or otherwise, without prior written permission from the publisher.

Malcom Rosenberg
370 N.W. 115 Way
Coral Springs, FL 3071
(954) 753-5915

Copyrighted 2001
Printed in the United States of America

INTRODUCTION

I have read patients' charts every working day for the past fifteen years. Reading the patient's chart is a nursing skill. It is as important as medication administration, sterile technique or therapeutic communication. Reading the chart is "knowing what's going on." It is knowing the patient's condition, labs, and doctors' orders.

The skill of reading charts is usually acquired on the job. This doesn't have to be the case. You can learn a lot right here, right now.

This book will have two parts: General guidelines for approaching the chart and reading illegible doctors' orders. First we'll look at reading handwriting.

Now almost all orders are handwritten. In a few years they'll be computerized. Many of the orders are barely legible. Reading these orders is a skill that can be learned with practice. This book begins that practice. I have included multiple examples of what I've seen to be the most frequent orders. I've written them every way I could, right handed, left handed, with my toes, printed, written, in every peculiar abbreviation and antiquated terminology.

All of these samples are fictitious. Any resemblance to actual patient orders is entirely coincidental.

clear liquid diet advance as
tolerated

coy pulled tomorrow 6:00am
O₂ 3 LT NC
daily pulse x-ray call < 92%
Hgb A1c
Acc ✓ 9/10
Δ all IV to PO
includes mixing meds
take off IV fluid bags
✓ SNF 7 A
Daily CXR
Cont esophagram R/o Aspiration
Keep HOB ↑ @ all times / Aspiration precautions
Wean 2 L O₂
Encourage cough, deep breathing, mobility status of reaction
Dialysis AM
Keep NPC

Page 2

$U winny 3 gm Q 6 hour
sures 2 An

200 cc sterile water through NGT Q 6h
SMA 18]
CBC] now

KCl 30 mEq in 150cc ½ WS over 3hr × 2 today

D/C Vasoxyn
Primaxin 500 IV 3g 8 hrs
Recheck K p̄ Replacement w/PB + call
Wean Levo off if tolerated day
Clonidine 0.1 PO BID
NTP " 96° (Keep SBP 120-150)
Norvasc Lyne 100 mg PO BID
    (Hold if SBP < 120)

Lanoxin 0.5 mg IV × 1
thorazine 25 mg PO Q 12°
Protein 375 mg PO QD
D/C N. th. probe
Inderal 60 mg po QD

CBC, SMA 18, ABG
& CXR in AM

Theophylline level in AM

Hold transfer. Keep in ICU

↓ Solumedrol to 50 mg IV push q 6 hrs

Zithromax 500 mg PO now
then 250 mg/day for 4 days

Complete PFT in AM

CBC SMA 18 - ABG
& CXR in AM

↑ Solumedrol to 60 mg IV q 6°
× 13 O 4 pm
Begin IV Aminophylline 500 mg in 500cc
D5W @ 20cc/hr
Spot O2 sat q AM × 2 dy

Postoperative Orders
Resume Preop Orders

Temp SR

OOB in chair with restraints

Jet Nebs with
0.3 cc pirbuterol
+ 3 cc NS Q6h

CBC c Diff

Dulcolax supp PR x 1 this AM
Colace 100mg po TID
Bedside commode

Transfer to rehab when DK & ortho

D/C Inderal
Start Norvasc 2.5 mg po qd.
Cardiology off case

D/C NTG paste
Nitropatch 0.4mg on AM off HS
Discharge today
D/C heplock

Admit to ICU
  Dx: pul emboli
      Hypoxemia
      ASHD
Cont fluids
VS routine
O₂ 2 L/m humidifier

Pyridoxine (Vit B₆) – 25 mg po qd
Pyridoxine (Vit B₆) – 25 mg po qd

PO₂ to 65mm – maintain SaO₂ > 92%

↑ Activity   Amb in Hall tid
                č assist

CT scan of the chest
  no contrast

Call Nursing Home
/Health again

Amitriptyline 10 mg po now for 1 dose
then 25 mg po HS daily

Remove non-crushing staples (R) thigh
D/C dressing
pack wound c̄ Betadine soaked strip
OK for D/C home tomorrow

Ambulate c̄ PT / gait training
Δ to Regular advance
Δc Acute CVA

Nursing please extubate
the pt @ 4h while awake
Consult "creation AV fistula (R) arm"
NPO p̄ MN except for PO meds c̄ sip of H₂O
may take Lanoxin Carafate Zantac on AM

Levaquin 500 mg po qd
Synthroid 0.175 g daily
Prograf 60 mg po daily
Lopressor 50 mg po BID
Lipitor 10 mg po daily
T. Cl.s 25 g po BID

Continue pulse ox
△ Hydralazine to q4°pm for SBP > 160 mmHg
Cardizem 30 mg po qid
D/C Pepcid
Start Prilosec 20 mg PO BID — email
  Biaxin 500 BID

Florinef 0.1 mg po daily — ?OK c̄ nephrology

Type + Xmatch 2 units packed RBC's & transfuse slowly
1 unit today, unit 4-28
H+H 4/28 after 2nd unit trans furd

Gastro Grafin enema early AM
Mag citrate 1/2 bottle tonight 8 PM
Dulcolol supp AM followed by
  fleet enema 7 AM

Stools for OB daily (x2)

Start Tube feeding

Nepro 3/4 Strenght → F.S. tomorrow
Rate 30cc/hr

↑ Head of bed 30°-45°

Hold if gastric residue is > 100cc

SMA-20
magnesium } tomorrow
CBC

All IV MEDS IN D5W
CBC SMA7 AM
Urine osmo + Na Day
Cycl Q 12h
Give 1 unit FFP with dialysis
PT PTT 6 PM

$1/2 NS @ 3gtt Q 6 hrs
CBC/ SMA7
  Jenny Bevcol ADA Diet
Berex 1mg PO QD
Glyburide 2.5mg PO QD
CARafgate SR. 90mg BID
HCL 0.1 5mg PO QD
Cogentin 3mg PO QD
Tylenol 650mg PO Q4 PRN
  for temp >101
old chart to the floor
Accuchek Q12hrs
If OK with Dr Smith Transfer
to telemetry
Up in Chair prn

Coumadin 10 mg PO Tonight
↑ Activity to OOB → chair with (L) leg elevated
Add TOD Bile to today's SMA 7
Call today's labs
↓ Diet to NAS 1800 Cal ADA
Begin Diabeta 2.5 mg PO QD
CT scan Abdomen + pelvis
PO contrast only No IV contrast
Call results

Coumadin 10 mg po today
Beginning now - PT QI and
call results for coumadin order

NPO until 3:00 pm Then clear liq
& if tolerate resume prior diet

Ancef 1 g IV
Demerol 50mg
Vistaril 4mg } IM on call
Robinul 0.2mg

Ativan 150mg } po on call
Reglan 10mg

D/C IV
D/C Accu
↑ Xanax to 0.5mg TID

Bld C/S x2 Q15 min
Stat CBC

Ophthalmology on call consult
Pulm de-?-

Stop ASA
Start Heparin drip at 100 u/h
PS, PTT now then Q8H
Give Heparin bolus 2500u IV after
initial PS, PTT are drawn, then start
the drip.

Adjust drip rate by 100u/hr increments
to keep PTT between 50-80
Call values to Dr. above

Hold Heparin
△ ECOTRIN 1 po QD
D/C TPTT
give ECOTRIN now

C&R SMA-7 in am
Dietary consult to try to ↑
  albumin
↑ Vasotec to 2.5 mg PO q 12h
if systolic BP > 98

Lopressor 25 mg PO stat and 25 mg PO BID

- SMA7 in AM
- CBC c Diff in AM, Manual diff
- Blood cultures x 2 — Now — 15 min apart
- Urine C&S tonight
- P. Chest X-ray in AM
- EKG in AM
- ID Consult S Dr Smith/Jones
- Admit - Monitor VS q1h x 4 then q4h Hep lock I & O BRP c BSC
- Nitropaste 1" q6h
- Norvasc 5 mg PO q am
- Diabeta 2.5 mg PO q am
- Daily EKG x 3
- Cardiac enzymes + Iso q 8h x 3
- SMA-7 daily x 3
- NTG 1/150 gr SL PRN for chest pain
- LOC PRN
- Tylenol ES 1 q 4h PRN
- O₂ by n/c at 3-4 L/min
- Arrhythmias Rx as per CCU protocol

- Ice packs ® wrist
- Velcro wrist splint
- Consciously off case:
- Kayexalate 30 g po now
- 1 oter 4 h p̄ above
- if K ≥ 5.5 repeat above Kayexalate
- add tid
- + fu te tebenctry postop

Haldol 0.5 mg i.m. q 8h prn
agitation   hold if sedated

Add CPK ī 50 ē mB band to labs
drawn in ER

Insert Foley Catheter
Urine for UA + C+S stat

Lanoxin 0.25 mg daily via PEG
Cardura 2 mg @ hs via PEG
Peri-Colace ī BID via PEG
    hold if diarrhea
Tylenol gr X-XV q 4 prn pain PEG)

Demerol 25 mg ē Phenergan 25 mg
im q 4h prn severe pain
Hold if sedated or confusion
            (   )

gastrograff?? BE Morning AM
no prep

Accuchecks ac + hs
0 - 60   OJ x2
61 - 200   No Rx
201 - 250   — 2u
251 - 300   4u   } Humulin R SQ
301 - 350   6u
351 - 400   8u
>400   — 10u

urine for cytology x2
renal U/S
DC foley in am?

roch urines x3
Motrin ? 600 prn
Chest spine CES result

may shower specimen C/o XT sections if needed

Trapeze on bed

IK Temp ≥ 100.5 f/u CXR
Blood cult 2 sets

SCRIBBLE TO ENGLISH TRANSLATION

Page 1

Clear liquid diet increase as tolerated
Chest X-ray portable tomorrow 6:00 a.m.
O2 3 liters nasal cannula
Daily pulse oxymetry call <92%
Hgb Htc
Accu check QID
Change all I.V. fluids to normal saline including mixing meds
Take all potassium from bags
Check SMA 7 in AM
Dailey chest X-ray
Cine esophogram rule out aspiration
Keep head of bed elevated at all times/ Aspiration precaution
Renew 2 liters O2
Encourage cough, deep breathing, mobilization of secretions
Dialysis A.M.
Keep NPO

Page 2

I.V. Unasyn 3 grams Q 6 hours
SMA 7 A.M.
200 cc sterile water through NGT Q 6 hours
SMA 18 CBC in A.M.
KCl 30 mEq in 150cc ½ NS over 3 hours times 2 today
D/C Unasyn
Primaxin 500 mg I.V. piggy back q 8 hours
Recheck potassium after replacement I.V. piggy back and call
Wean off nipride drip
Clonidine 0.1 p.o. B.I.D.
Nitro paste 1" Q 6 hours (Keep SBP 120-150)
Normadyne 100mg P.O. B.I.D. (Hold systolic blood pressure < 120)
Lanoxin 0.5 mg X 1
Tenormin 25 mg P.O. Q 12 hours
Ecotrin 325 mg P.O. Q day

D/C nitro paste
Imdur 60 mg P.O. Q day

Page 3

CBC, SMA 8 ABG
Chest x-ray in A.M.
Theophylline level in A.M.
Hold transfer keep in ICU
Decrease solumedrol to 50mg I.V. push q 6 hours
Zithromax 500mg PO now then 250mg/day for 4 days
Complete pulmonary function test in AM
CBC SMA 18 chest x-ray in AM in AM (they duplicate a lot)
Increase solumedrol to 60mg IV q 6 hours
Head of bed at 45degrees
Begin IV aminophylline 500mg in 500cc D5W @ 20cc/hr
Spot O2 saturation q AM x 2 days

Page 4

Postoperative Orders
Resume Previous Orders
Home A.M.
Out of bed in chair with restraints
Jet Neb with 0.3 cc proventil + 3 cc normal saline Q 6 hours
CBC with dif
Dulcolax suppository P.R. X 1 this A.M.
Colace 100 mg P.O. T.I.D.
Bedside Commode
Transfer to rehab when o.k. with ortho
D/C Inderal
Start Norvasc 2.5 mg P.O. Q day
Cardiology off case
D/C nitro paste
Nitro patch 0.4 mg on A.M. off H.S.
Discharge today
D/C Hep Lock

Admit to ICU
Dx pulmonary emboli hypotension ASHD
Condition fair
Vital Signs routine
O2 2 liters/min
Pyridoxine (vit B6) 25mg PO QID or QD?
Increase O2 to 6 liters/min Maintain saturation > 92%
Change activity Ambulate in hall tid with assist
CT scan of the chest No contrast
Call nursing home health agency
Amitriptyline 10mg. PO Now for one dose then 25 mg. PO HS Daily

Remove remaining staples right thigh
D/C dressing
Paint wound with betadine swab tid
OK for d/c home tomorrow
Ambulate with PT/gait training
Change to regular admit
Diagnosis acute CVA
Nursing please ambulate the patient Q4h while awake
consent "creation AV fistula right arm"
NPO past midnight except for PO meds with sips of H2O
May take lanoxin carafate zantac in A.M.

Levaquin 500 mg. po QD
Synthroid 0.175 mg. Daily (no mention of PO but everything else is)
Prozac 60 mg. Po daily
Lopressor 50 mg. Po BID
Lipitor 10 mg. Po daily
Ticlid 25 mg. Po BID
Continue pulse oxymeter
Change hydralazine to q4h prn for systolic blood pressure >160 hg
Cardizem 30 mg. Po QID
D/C Pepcid
Start Prilosec PO BID with meals
Biaxin 500 with meals (it doesn't say mg.)
Florinef 0.1 mg. PO daily if OK with nephrology
Type and cross mstch 2 units of packed red blood cells and transfuse slowly
1 unit 4-28
H&H 4-28 after 2nd unit transfused
Gastrografin enema early AM
Mag citrate ½ bottle tonight 8 PM
Dulcolax suppository (7 AM written below) AM followed by fleets enema

Stool for occult blood daily times two
Insert tube feeding
Nepro ¾ strength Full strength tomorrow
Rate 30 cc/hr
Raise Head of bed 30 to 45 degrees
Hold if gastric residue is > 100cc
SMA 20, magnesium, CBC tomorrow
All I.V. meds in D5W
CBC SMA 7 in A.M.
Urine osmolarity and sodium today
Lytes Q 12 hours
Give one unit fresh frozen plasma with dialysis
PT PTT 6P.M.

Page 9

I.V. Unasyn 3 grams q 6 hours
CBC/SMA 7
2 gram sodium 1800 cal ADA diet (the first word is difficult but it would have to pertain to diets)
Bumex 1 mg. PO QD
Glyburide 2.5 mg. PO QD
Cardizem SR 90 mg. BID (sustained release is a tablet or PO)
Haldol 5 mg. PO QD
Cogentin 3 mg. PO QD
Tylenol 650 mg. PO QID PRN for temp > 101
Old chart to the floor
Accu check QID (This is hard. QD or QID? It couldn't hurt to do it AC & HS, or QID)
If OK with Dr. Smith transfer to telemetry
Up in chair in AM

Page 10

Coumadin 10 mg. PO tonight
Change activity to out of bed to chair with leg elevated
Add total and direct billi to today's SMA 7
Call today's labs
Change diet to no added salt 1800 ADA
Begin diabeta 2.5 mg. PO QD
CT scan abdoman and pelvis
PO contrast only only no I.V. contrast
Call results
Coumadin 10 mg. PO today
Beginning now PT QD and
Call results for coumadin order

Page 11

NPO until 3:00 then sips H2O (water)
& if tolerated renew previous diet
NPO after midnight
Demerol 50 mg. I.M on call
Versed 4 mg. I.M. on call

Robinol 0.2 mg. I.M. on call
Axid 150 mg. PO on call
Reglan 10 mg. PO on call
D/C IVF (I.V. fluids)
D/C Ancef
Increase Xanax to 0.5 mg. TID
Blood culture and sensitivity times two Q 15 minutes
Stat CBC
Ophthalmology on call consult (consult the ophthalmologist on call)
Pulmonary isolation

Stop aspirin
Start heparin drip at 100 units/hour
PT/PTT now then Q 8 hours
Give heparin bolus 2500 units I.V. after
Initial PT/PTT are drawn, then start the drip
Adjust drip rate by 100 units/hour increments
To keep PTT between 50 and 80
Call neuro to OK above
Hold heparin
Change ecotrin 1 PO Q 6
D/C PT PTT
Give ecotrin now
Chest x-ray SMA 7 in AM
Dietary consult to try to increase albumin
Increase Vasotec to 2.5 mg PO Q 12 hours
If systolic blood pressure > 98

Lopressor 25 mg PO stat and 25 mg. PO BID
SMA 7 in AM
CBC with Diff manual Manual diff
Blood cultures times 2 – now - 15 minutes apart
Urine C and S tonight
Portable chest x-ray in AM
EKG in AM
ID (infectious disease) consult Dr. Smith/Jones

Admit monitor Vital signs q 1 hour times 4 then
Q 4 hours hep lock intake and output bedrest with bathroom privileges
Nitropasst 1" Q 6 hours
Norvasc 5 mg. Q AM
Diabeta 2.5 mg. PO Q AM
Daily EKG times 3
Cardiac enzymes + iso's q 8 hours times 3
SMA 7 daily times 3
Nitroglycerine 1/150 grain sl (sublingual) PRN for chest pain
LOC PRN (laxative of choice)
Tylenol ES (extra strength) 1 q 4 hours PRN
O2 by nasal canula at 3-4 liters/min
Arrhythmia treatment per CCU protocol

Ice packs left wrist
Velcro wrist splint
Cardiology off case
Kayexolate 30 grams PO now
Lytes 4 hours after above
If k greater than or equal to 5.5 repeat above Kayexolate
Hold ticlid
Transfer to telemetry postop
Haldol 0.5 mg I.M. q 8 hours prn
Agitation hold if sedated
Add CPK Iso with MB band to labs
Drawn in ER
Insert foley catheter
Urine for UA + C / S stat
Lanoxin 0.25 mg. Daily via PEG
Cardura 2 mg. @ HS via PEG
Pericolace one BID via PEG
Hold if diarrhea
Tylenol gr X-XV (10-15 grains, 650-975 mg., two-three tablets)
Demerol 25 mg. With Phenergan 25 mg.
I.M. q 4 hours prn severe pain
Hold if sedated or increased confusion

Gastrograffin barium enema Monday AM
No prep
Accuchecks ac + hs
0 - 60   O.J. x 2
61 – 200 No Rx
201 – 250 2 units
251 - 300 4 units   Humulin R SQ
301 – 350 6 units
351 – 400 8 units
> 400   10 units

urine for cytology X 2
renal ultra sound
D/C foley in AM &
Rack urine X 3
maintain 2 liters/min prn
chart sputum C&S result
may obtain specimen via nasogastric suction if
needed
trapeze on bed
if temp greater than or equal to 100.5 get chest x-ray X 1
blood culture 2 sets

LAB RESULTS & DOCTORS' ORDERS

From my experience, there are three different ways (and times of the day) to look at a chart: #1 The first is on admission when the patient has not been in the room for more than an hour. Most of what you know is from the emergency room report or what the patient has told you. At this point there is only the initial set of orders and the ER labs. You are mainly looking for abnormal labs, important medications that you have to give right away (and probably go up to pharmacy to get). You will probably have to get lab results from the computer. It is a good idea to print them and put them on the chart. I remember one chest pain admission when the ER gave me an essentially negative report. In fact the enzymes were positive with S-T elevations and the patient was in the middle of a heart attack. All lab values that are back should be checked. All of the admitting orders should be checked.

Depending on the admitting diagnosis labs would be checked differently over the course of the day. If the diagnosis is chest pain then cardiac enzymes should be anticipated. You should make a note of what needs to be done and when. You might ask the secretary what the times are for the second and third set of enzymes are to be drawn. If the patient is in CHF and taking diuretics you'll be watching potassium levels. If the patient is in with G.I. bleed you'll be watching the H&H and anticipating the next blood draw.

#2 The second situation is during the course of a busy day. Here you'll be checking the labs as they come in and the orders as they are written. If you see your patient's doctor has just written orders, it is a good idea to check the chart and make sure the orders are clear and legible (sometimes they're not). It's a lot easier to nab the doctor on the spot to clarify an order you can't read.

#3 The third situation is at night when the 24 hour chart check is usually done. At three in the morning you're checking to see that everything was done. That's orders entered, blood drawn, x-rays done, results obtained, consents signed, consults called, etc. You are doing the same thing as they did on day shift but with fewer distractions.

PROGRESS NOTES AND HISTORY & PHYSICAL

The best way to find out about your patient is to read the doctors' progress notes, the history & physical and the consultation sheets. The history and physical is usually dictated, transcribed and typed. That's great. But it takes a day or two to get on the chart. Reading progress notes is very difficult. I can barely read them. In reading orders you know what to expect... "CBC, SMA 7 chest x-ray in AM". But progress notes are a whole different vocabulary.

There are two instances where you will need to read them. When an abnormal lab value or condition appears, the question is whether to call the doctor. At 2:00 A.M. that's a very big question. To see if the doctor knows about it, you'd look in the progress notes. They usually note pertinent labs. They might say it in less specific words like hyperkalemia or hyponatremia.

The other instance where I've had to comb through the progress notes is clearance for surgery. They sometimes say it very quietly like, "surgery ok." I've always thought that should be an order. On the surgical checklist I always write the date next to my initials.

TIPS

Make sure the order sheets are stamped with the right patients. You usually assume the chart has the correct stamps. A wrong name on the sheet would result in a very serious med error. Also check that the correct patient's EKG is in your patient's chart.

Another good idea is to make a list of doctors' signatures in the format on the next page. That will help you figure out who wrote the orders.

Doctor Signature List

Signature	Name
signature	Dr Adams
signature	Dr Anderson
signature	Dr James Anderson
signature	Dr Benton
signature	Dr Robert Burns
signature	Dr Robert Bailey
signature	Dr Carrino
signature	Dr Michael Douglas

For Students...For L.P.N.s...For R.N.s...

DRUG CALCULATIONS FOR NURSES WHO HATE NUMBERS
by MALCOLM ROSENBERG, R.N.

IF YOU HAVE TROUBLE WITH DRUG CALCULATIONS, THESE CARICATURES COULD BE YOUR FRIENDS

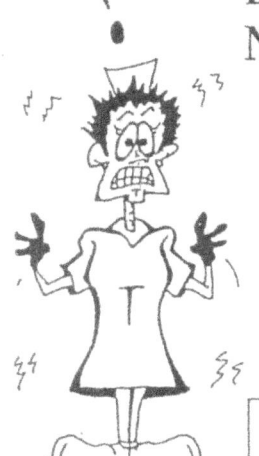

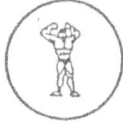 30 mg 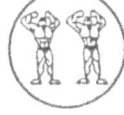 60 mg 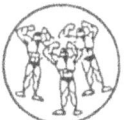 90 mg

Viagra Simplified
Understanding the Erection

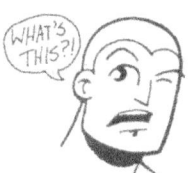

To get more information and order online: www.simplifiednursing.com
or send a check or money order made out to:
Malcolm Rosenberg • P.O. Box 770793 • Coral Springs, FL 33077 • (954) 753-5915

NAME_____ E-MAIL_____
ADDRESS_____
CITY_____ STATE_____ ZIP_____

Drug Calculations For Nurses Who Hate Numbers	$18.95	☐
Simplified Cardiac Medications	$18.95	☐
Simplified Arterial Blood Gases	$18.95	☐
Hemodynamics	$11.95	☐
Simplified Ventilators	$7.95	☐
Heart Sounds Simplified	$7.95	☐
Simplified Blood Clotting	$6.95	☐ TOTAL
Improved Chart Reading Skills	$3.95	☐ ENCLOSED $_____
Viagra Simplified	$6.95	

MORE GREAT BOOKS!

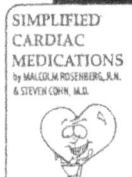
SIMPLIFIED CARDIAC MEDICATIONS
by MALCOLM ROSENBERG, R.N. & STEVEN COHN, M.D.

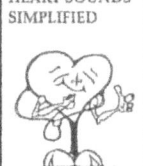
SIMPLIFIED ARTERIAL BLOOD GASES

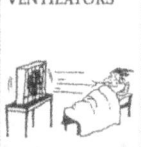
HEART SOUNDS SIMPLIFIED

SIMPLIFIED VENTILATORS

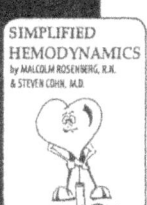
IMPROVED CHART READING SKILLS

SIMPLIFIED HEMODYNAMICS
by MALCOLM ROSENBERG, R.N. & STEVEN COHN, M.D.

For more infomation write or call: **MALCOLM ROSENBERG • P.O. BOX 770793 • CORAL SPRINGS, FL 33077 • (954) 753-5915**
and PLEASE VISIT OUR WEBSITE AT: **www.simplifiednursing.com**

Improve Your Chart Reading Skills ©2001   Retail: $3.95

www.ingramcontent.com/pod-product-compliance
Lightning Source LLC
Chambersburg PA
CBHW081812170526
45167CB00008B/3411